Copyright

Total Transformation Health Solutions LLC.
www.transformedhealth.org

Brianna L. Mosby, BS, PharmD
Registered Pharmacist AFPA Certified Holistic Nutritionist

Publisher's Note: This is a work of non-fiction for educational purposes only. The information included is not medical advice. Before making any changes in your diet or lifestyle, be sure to consult with a medical professional.

Photographer: Riddell T. Gardner, Sr. (Gardner Innovations)

Book Layout © 2023 Alexis M. Creative Agency LLC.

Dr. Bri's Blends Smoothie Guide/ Dr. Brianna Mosby

ISBN: 9798850113889
Imprint:
Independently published

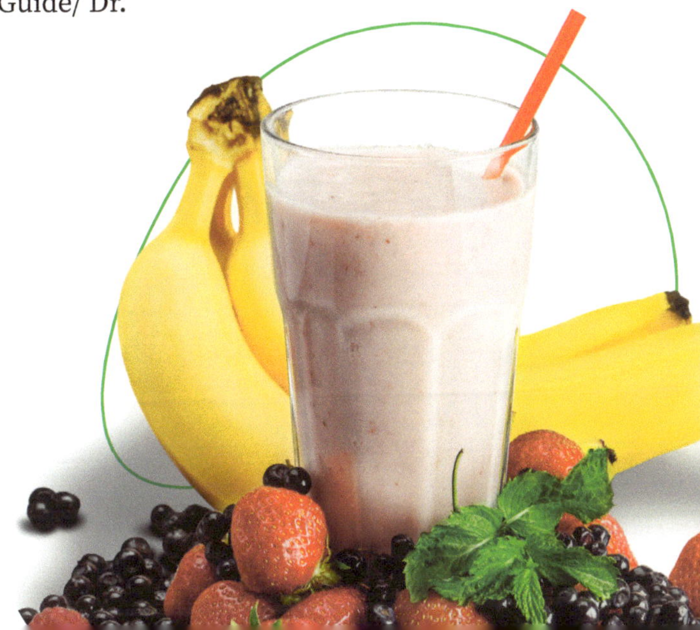

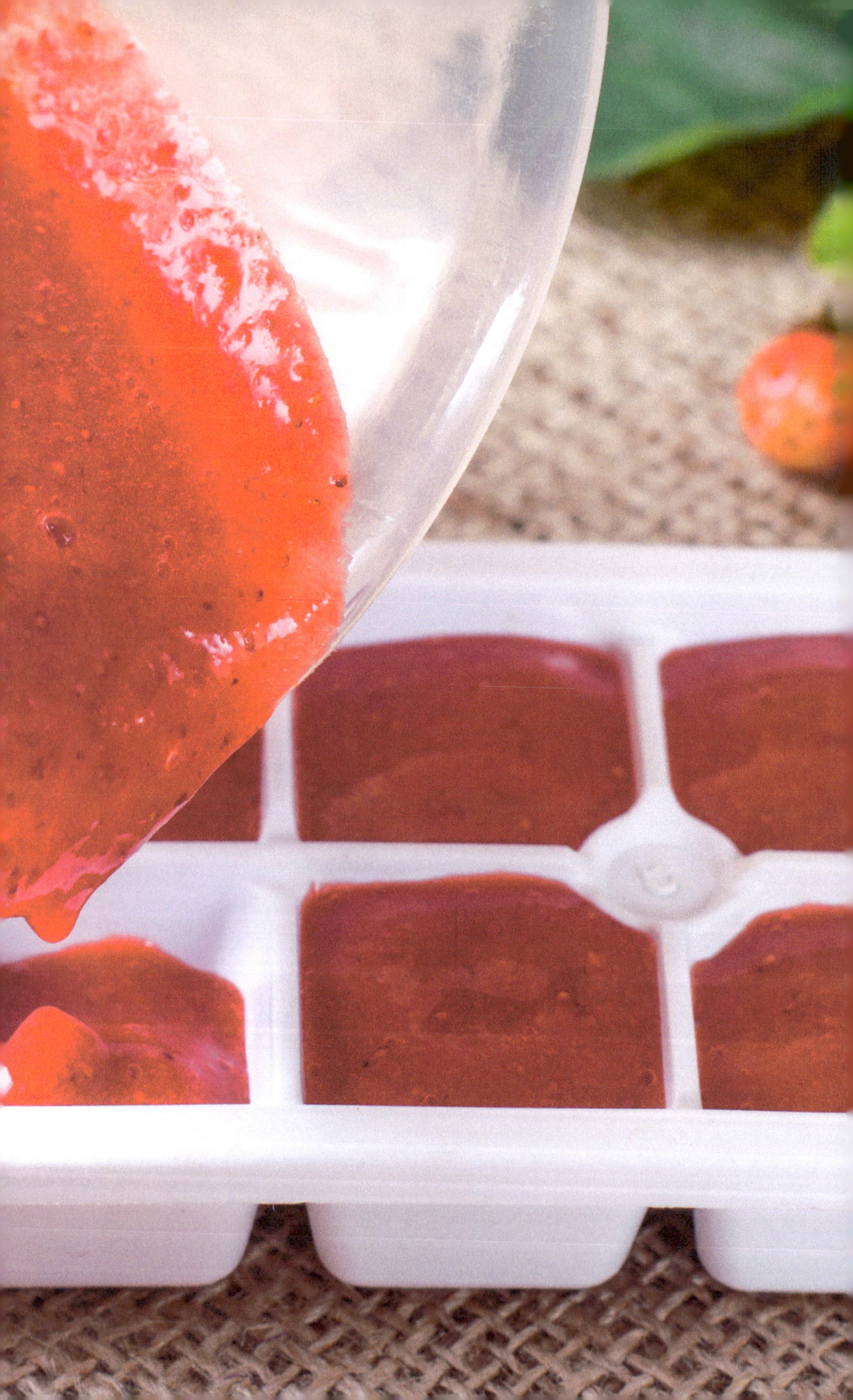

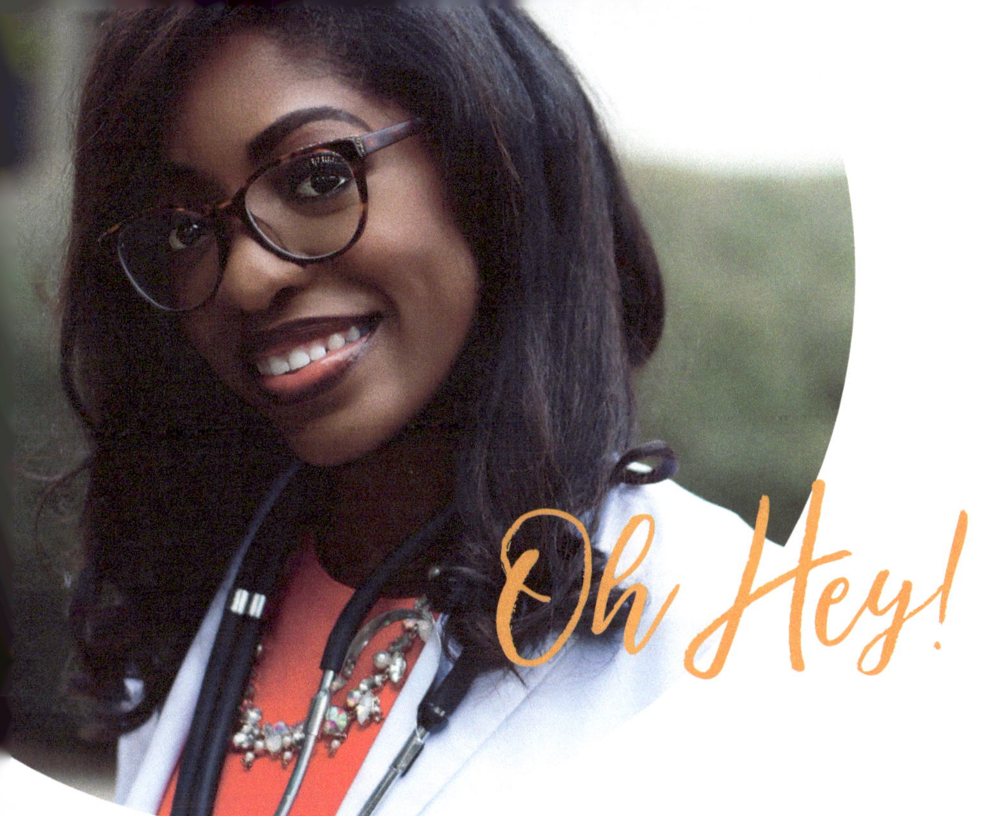

I see you -- making better choices and choosing to continue your daily discovery of what's best for you.

Health & wellness is not a one-size fits all model. What works for one, does not always work for the other. And you know what? That's okay! As you continue to grow and evolve, first things first:

- **Being honest** with yourself. Set goals that are attainable and sustainable.

- **Grace.** Extend yourself as much as you need as often as you need.

- You have to **put in the work** but remember not to neglect the resources in the circle surrounding you.

Know, above all else, I am rooting for you. Thank you so very much for your support. I look forward to helping you in your continued journey.

In Your Corner,

Dr. Bri

Much like the arguably convenient use of a daily multivitamin, smoothies serve as a great on-the-go option to contribute to your dietary needs.

Diversifying your diet is imperative to optimizing the absorption of the vitamin spectrum.

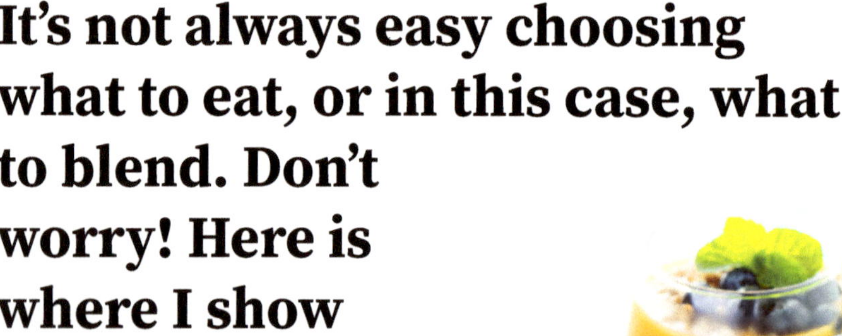

Without sufficient vitamin intake, risk of deficiencies arise, resulting in potential vision & skin changes, anemia, bone irregularities, nerve & muscle challenges, and more.

It's not always easy choosing what to eat, or in this case, what to blend. Don't worry! Here is where I show up for you.

This smoothie guide is designed to equip you with the necessary framework to make deciding a bit easier.

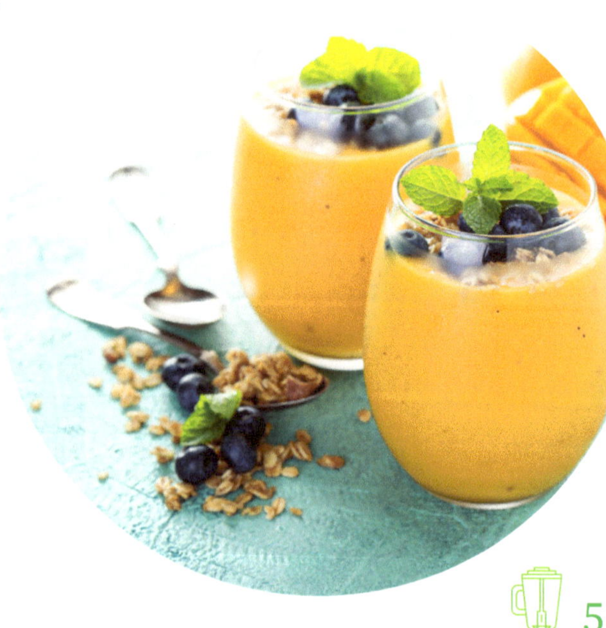

Let's get into it!

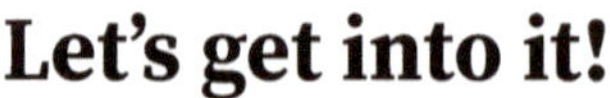

The Goodies Inside

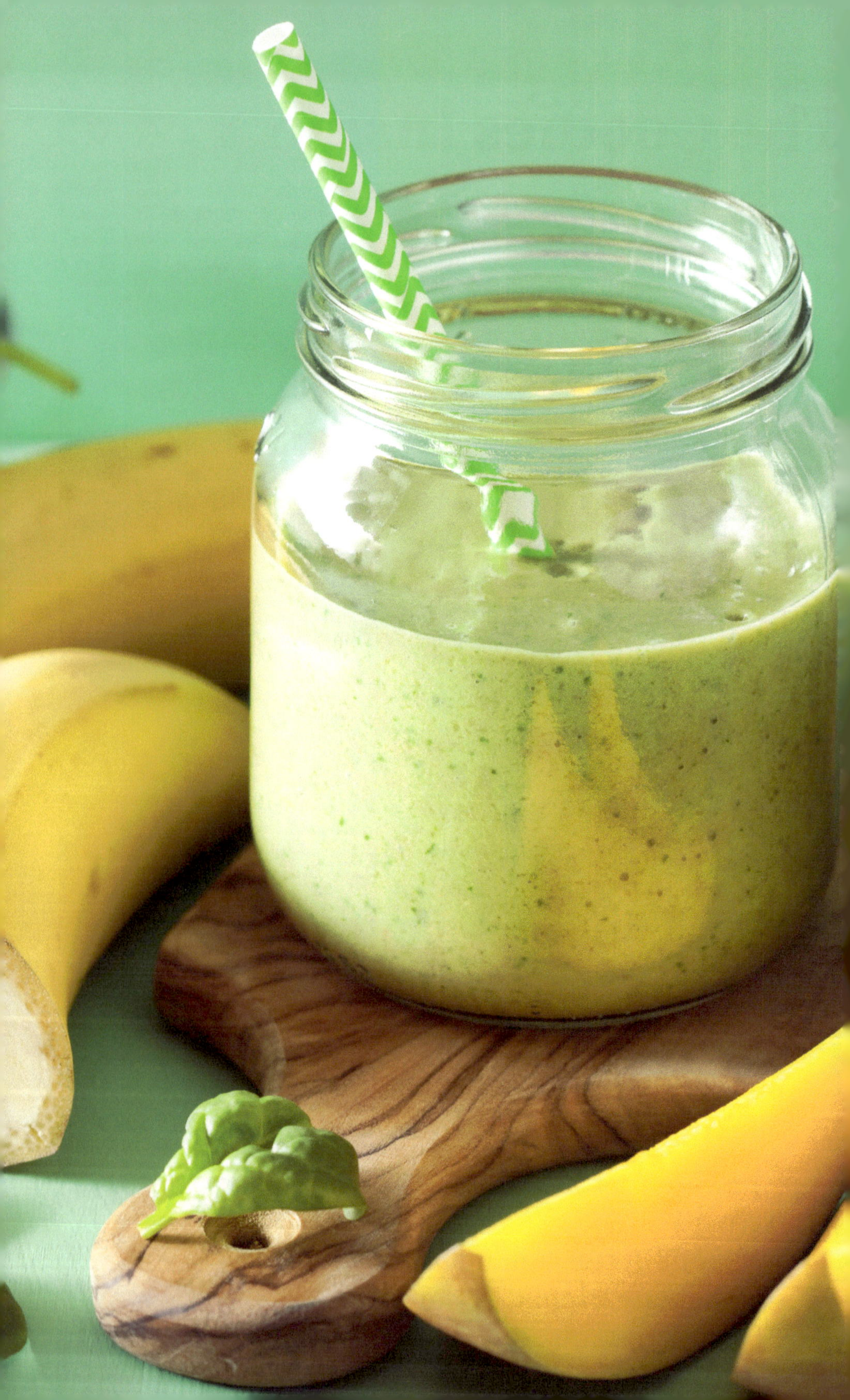

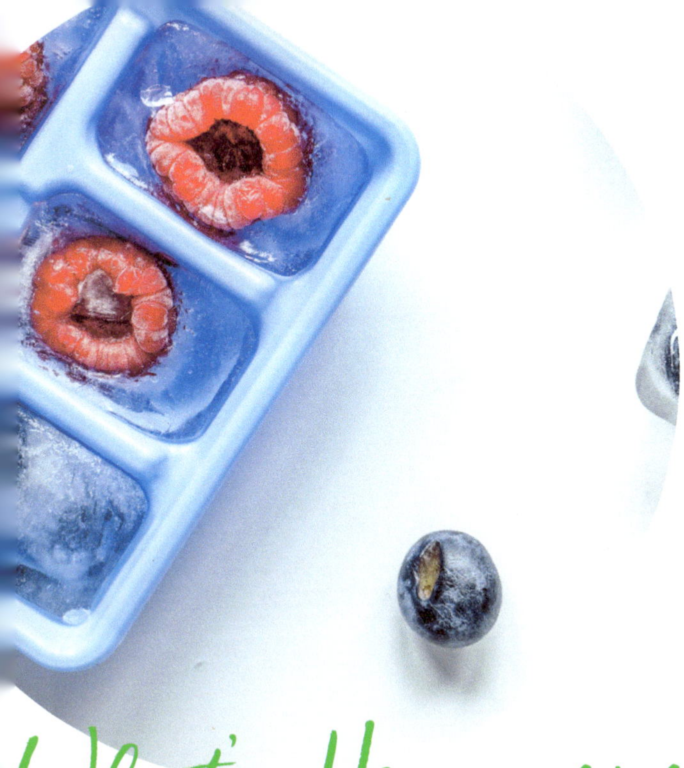

What's Happening

Inside of your body

The next few pages will uncover your
Symptoms + Potential Deficiency = Food Solutions

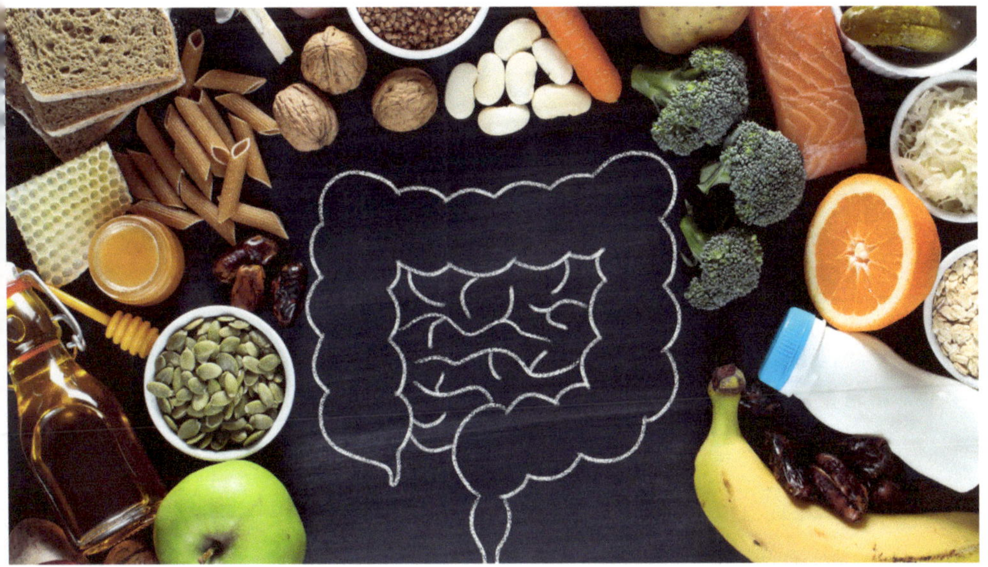

Symptoms

Dry skin
Frequent colds
Frequent infections
Poor night vision

Potential Deficiency
Vitamin A

Add Me in Your Blends

Carrots
Tomatoes
Beets
Apples
Pears

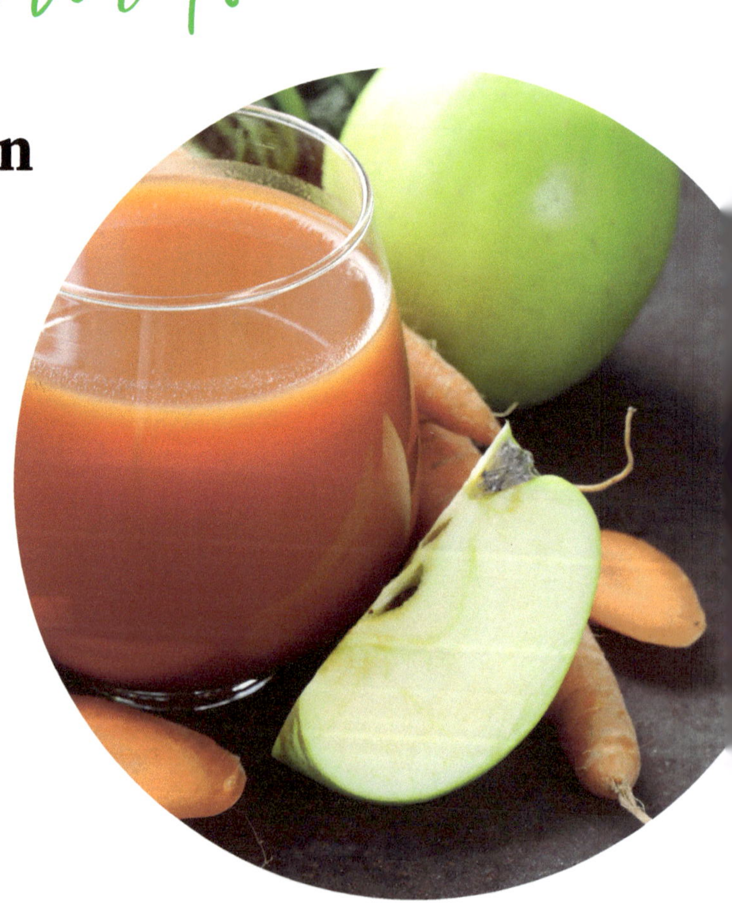

Symptoms

Muscle pain
Poor concentration
Headaches
Lack of energy
Poor appetite

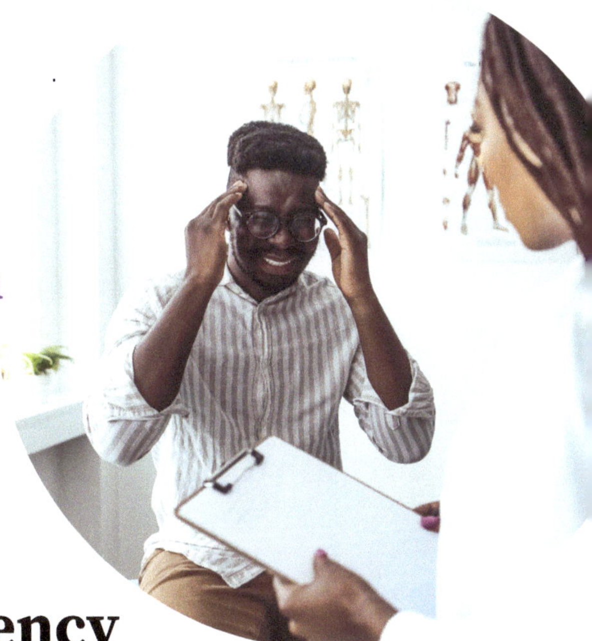

Potential Deficiency
B Vitamins

Add Me in Your Blends

Bananas
Avocado
Beets
Yogurt
Oatmeal

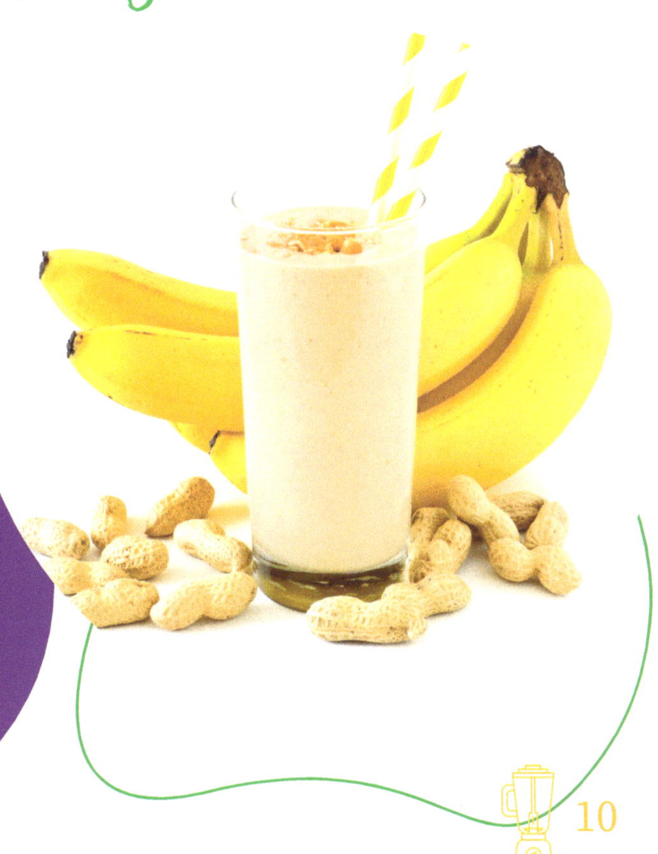

Symptoms

Aches & pains
Nosebleeds
Frequent colds or
infections
Easy bruising

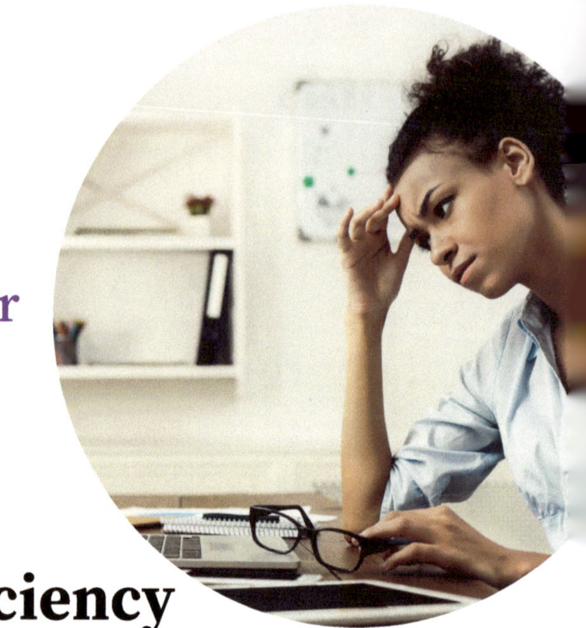

Potential Deficiency
Vitamin C

Add Me in Your Blends

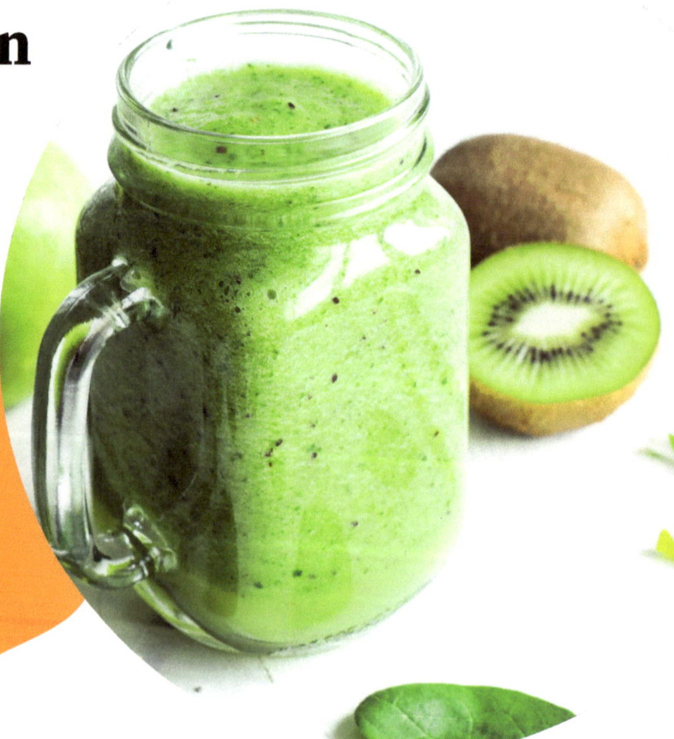

Oranges
Mangos
Tomatoes
Strawberries
Lemons
Kiwifruits

Symptoms

Fatigued
Irritable
Anxious
Depressed
Backaches

Potential Deficiency

Vitamin D

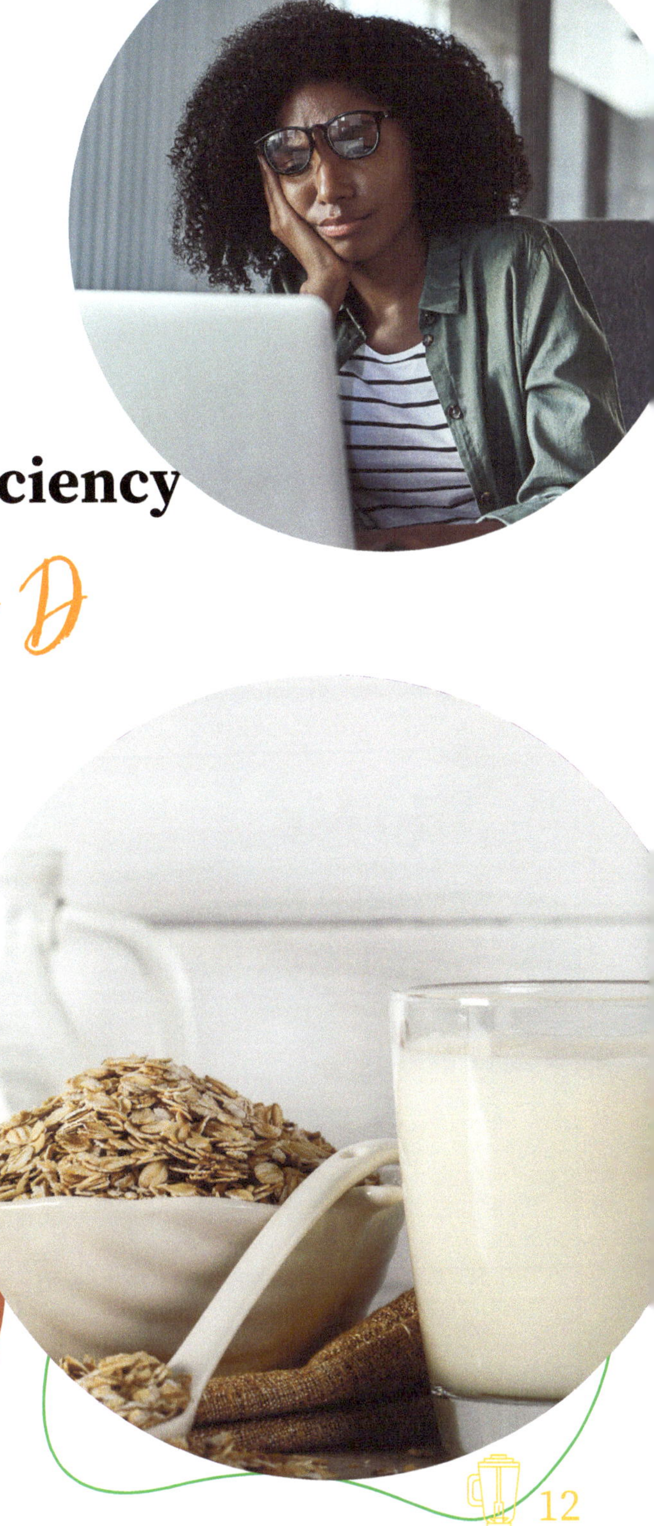

Add Me in Your Blends

Oat Milk
Almond Milk
Orange Juice

Symptoms

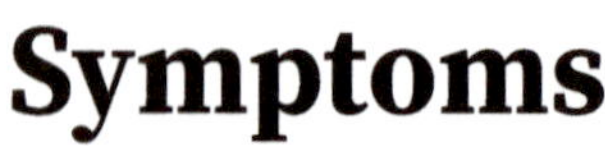

Exhaustion after exercising
Reduced libido
Easy bruising
Slow wound healing

Potential Deficiency

Vitamin E

Add Me
in Your
Blends

Spinach
Avocado
Almonds
Peanut Butter

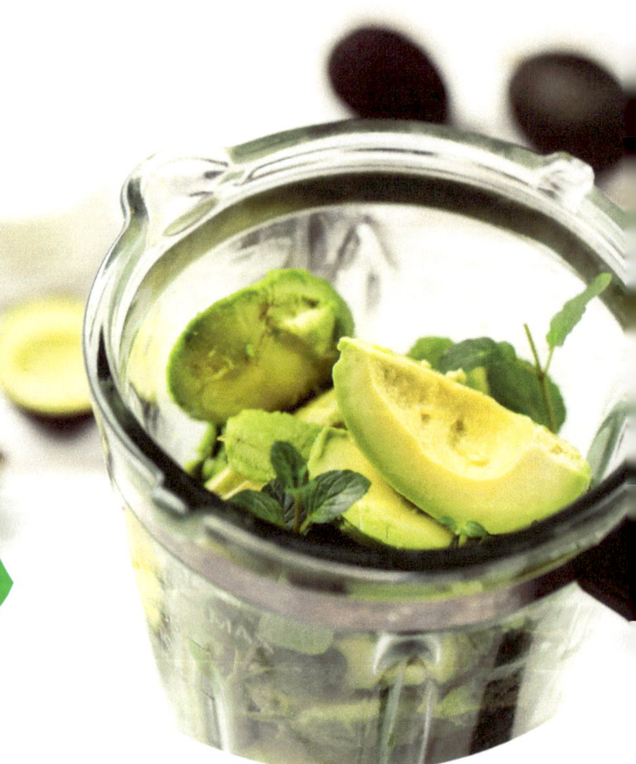

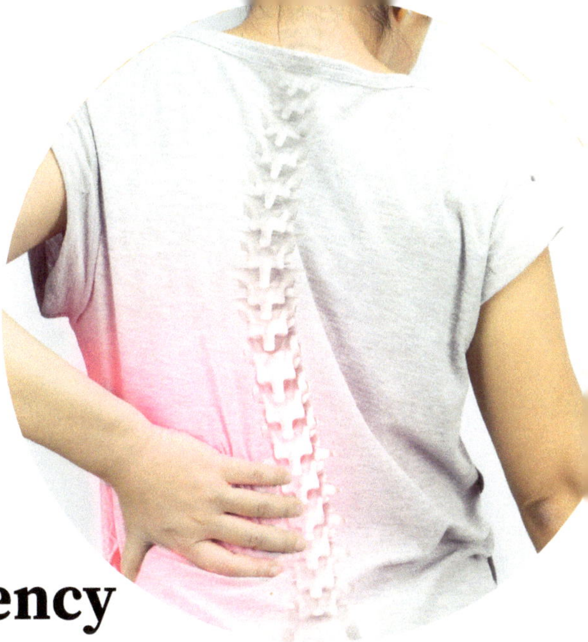

Symptoms

Brittle bones
Slow clotting
after a cut

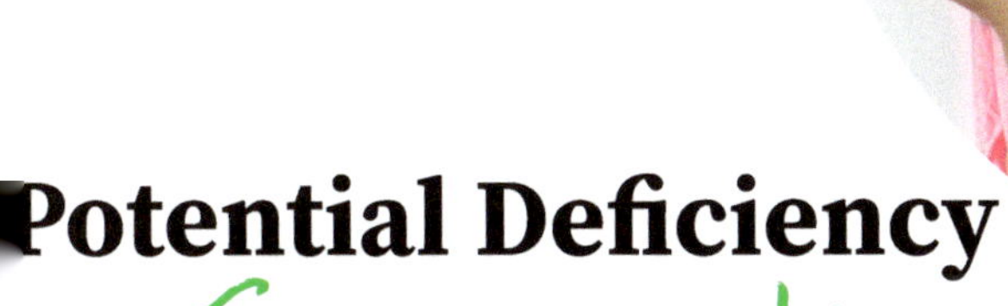

Potential Deficiency

Vitamin K

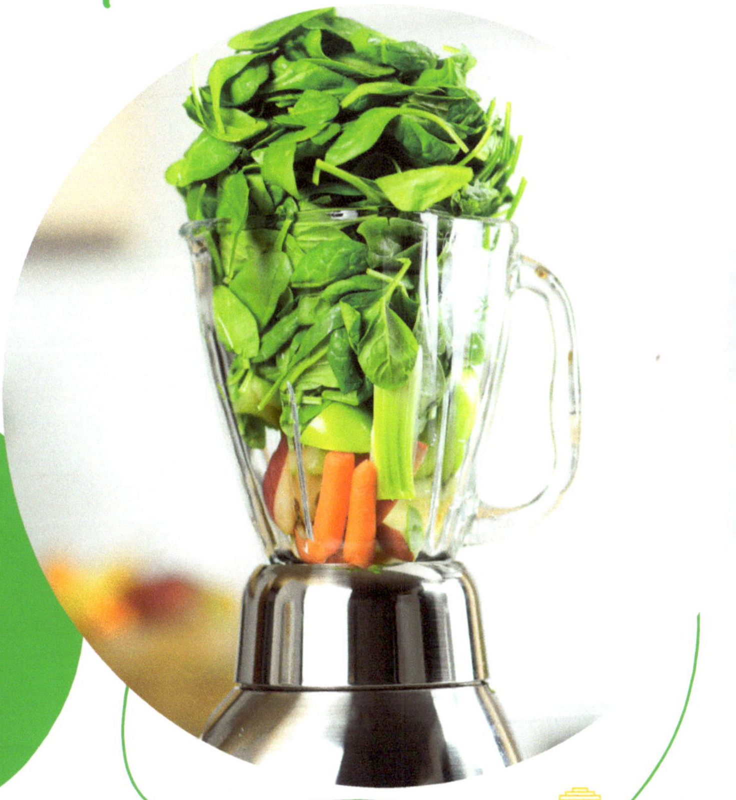

Add Me in Your Blends

Green, leafy vegetables
Carrots

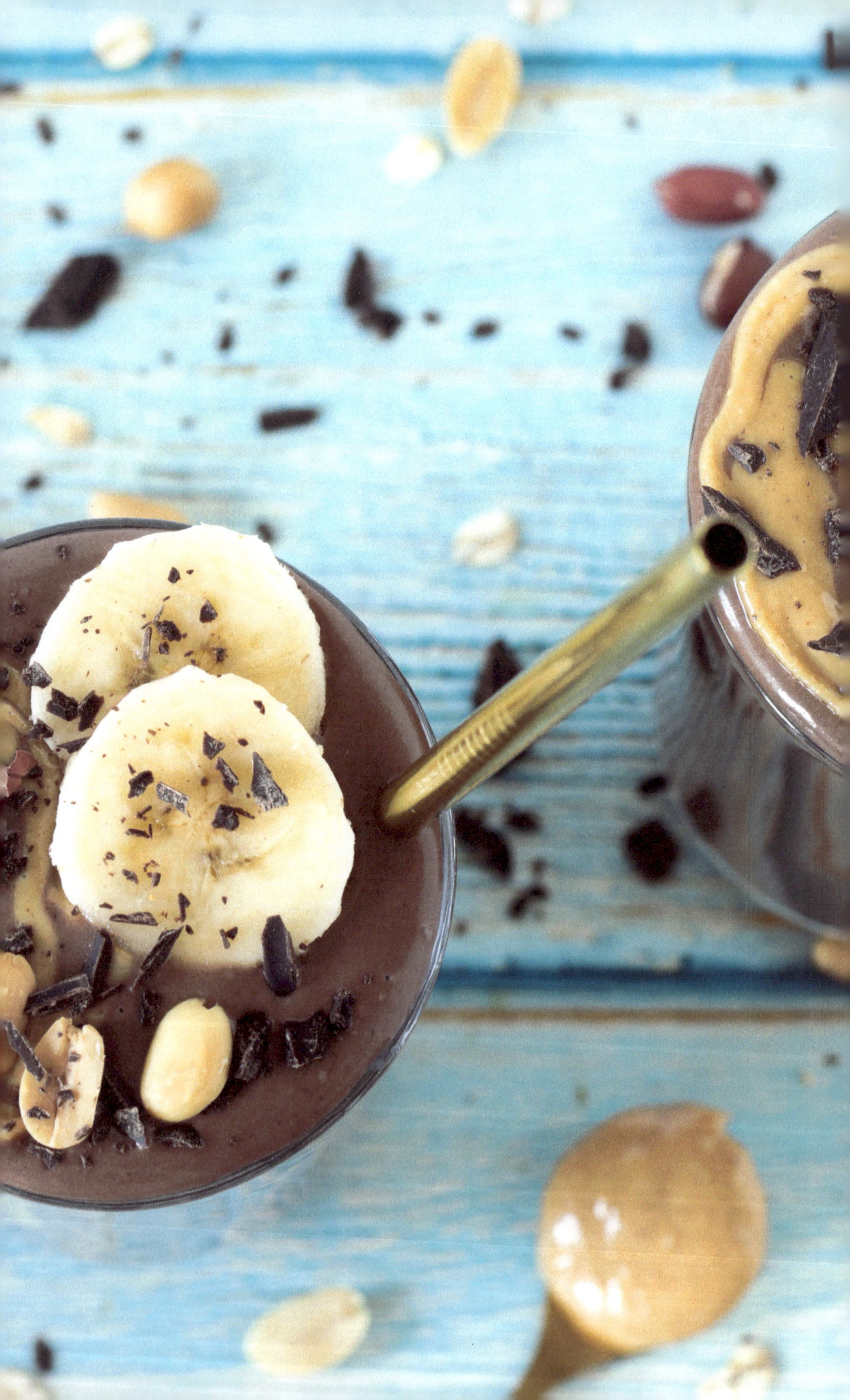

What's In Dr. Bri's Blends

Categorized based on the predominant vitamin content.

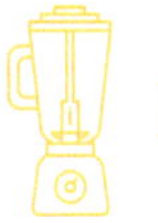

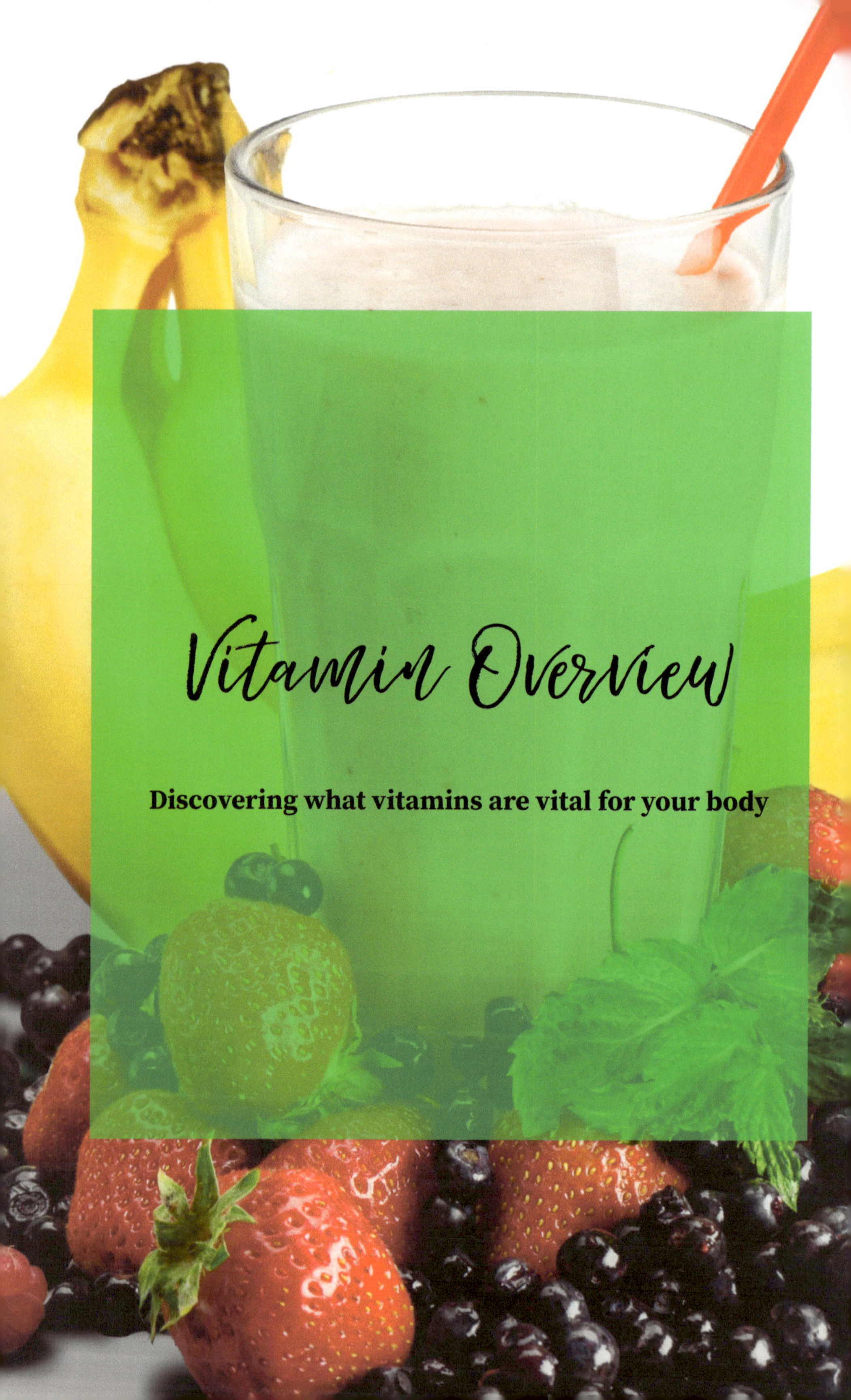
Vitamin Overview
Discovering what vitamins are vital for your body

Vitamins in Food

Vitamin D
Egg yolks
Fish
Fish oil & cod liver oil
Fortified dairy products
Fortified orange juice
Mushrooms

Vitamin A
Cantaloupe
Carrots
Green leafy vegetables
Pumpkin
Sweet potatoes
Dairy products
Eggs
Red peppers

B Vitamins
Non-citrus fruits
Potatoes
Seafood
Dairy products
Eggs
Poultry
Avocados
Whole grains
Nuts

Vitamin E
Nuts
Seeds
Vegetable oils
Mango
Kiwifruit

Vitamin C
Fruit
(citrus & non-citrus)
Juices
(fruit & vegetable)
Broccoli
Brussel sprouts
Peppers
Tomatoes

Vitamin K
Green vegetables
Spinach
Kale
Turnip &
Collard greens

*While these are not all inclusive lists, it's a great way to find a starting point to enhance your intake.

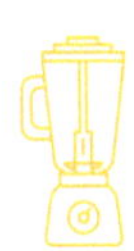

18

Water-Soluble Vitamins

Dissolved in the water in your body.

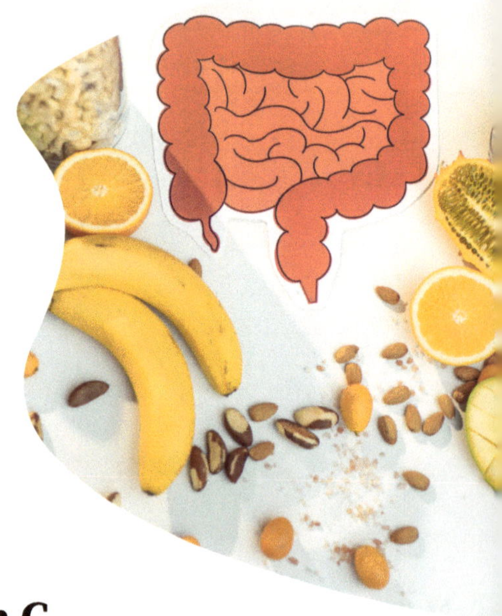

Vitamin B Complex

Collectively they aid in:

- Immune function
- Nervous System function
- Red blood cell formation
- Conversion of food into energy
- Overall health

Vitamin C

- Antioxidant
- Collagen & connective tissue formation
- Immune function
- Wound healing
- Helps the body absorb iron & folic acid

There are (8) B vitamins comprising the complex, all working together to maximize the effects of each other.

Fat-Soluble Vitamins

...bsorbed with the fats we consume.

VITAMIN A

Supports healthy eyesight & immune system functions
Contributes to growth & development
Important for red blood cell formation
Skin health

Vitamin D

Vital for bone health, growth & calcium balance; muscle & nerve function
Provides immune system support, aiding in combating bacteria & viruses
Blood pressure regulation
Hormone production
Controls calcium absorption

Vitamin E

- Antioxidant
- Contributes to blood cell formation
- Immune function
- Reduces menopause symptoms
- Anticoagulant

Vitamin K

- Essential for blood clotting
- Strengthens bones

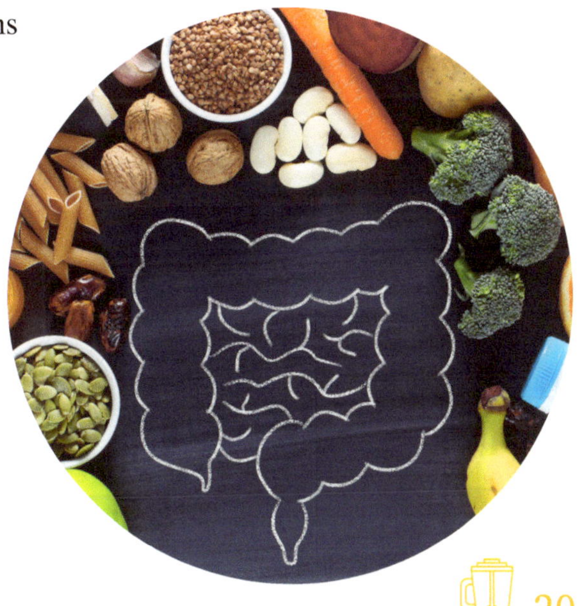

Fun fact:

Your gut is where Vitamin K is made.

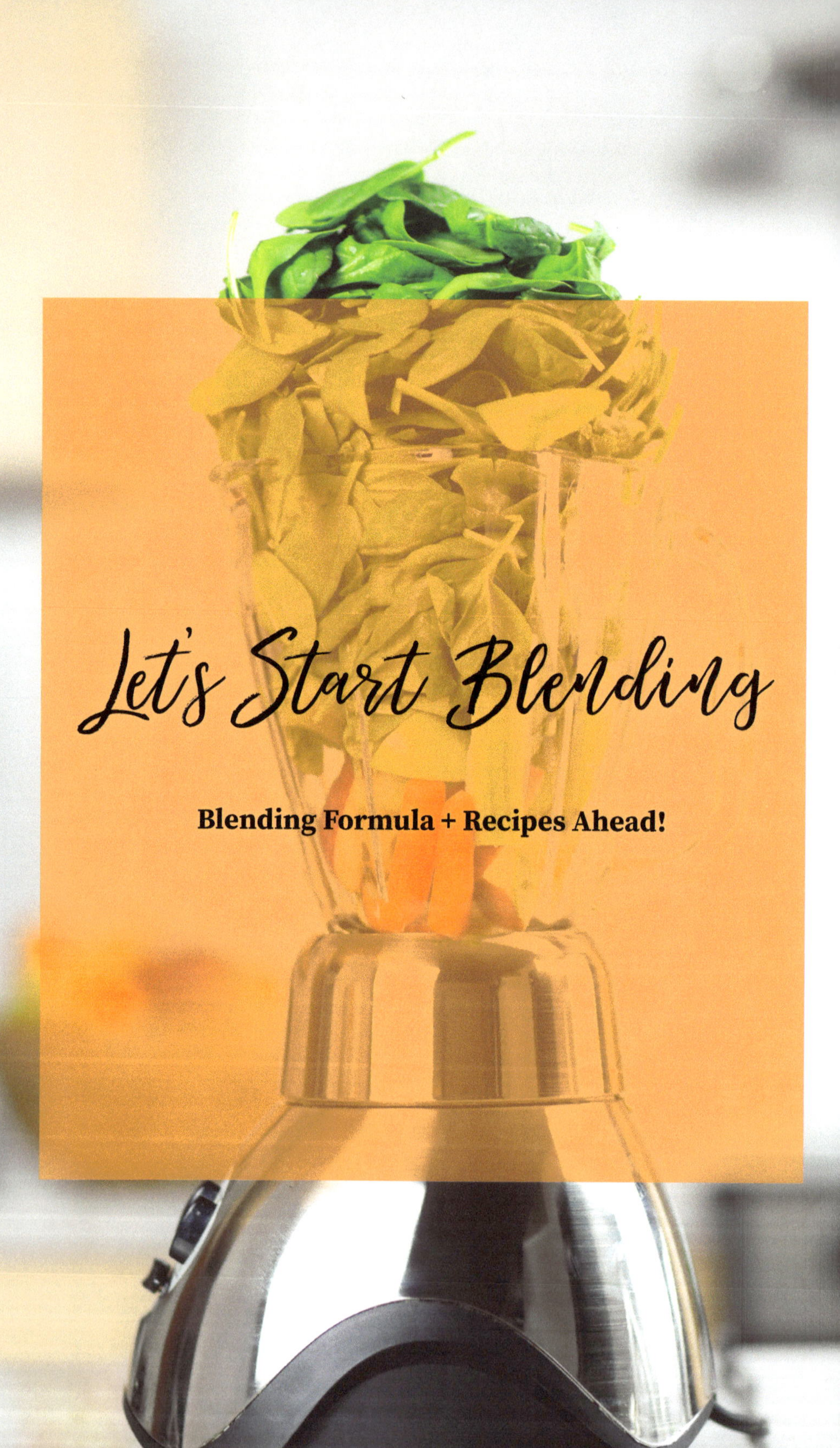

Let's Start Blending
Blending Formula + Recipes Ahead!

Build Your Blend

Select a Liquid Base:

Fruit Juice (100%)
Vegetable Juice (100%)
Plant Based Milk (Almond, Cashew, Oatmilk)

Choose Your Add-In(s):

Fruits
Vegetables
Spices (cinnamon, turmeric, ginger)
Herbs (mint, lavender, rosemary)
Creatine & Protein Powders

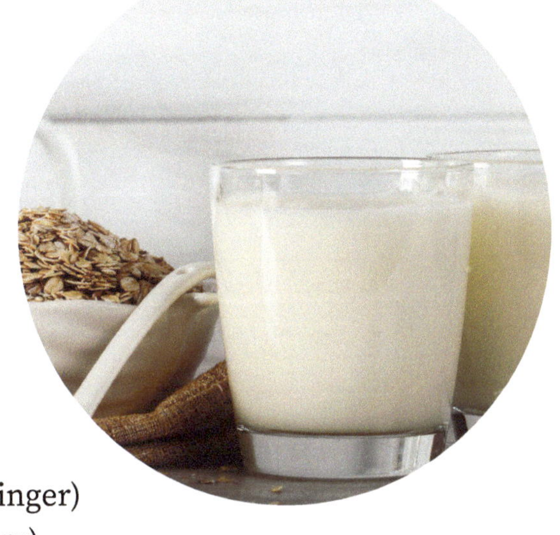

Consistency Adjustments:

For thicker smoothies
Frozen fruit/vegetables
Greek yogurt
Avocado
Chia seeds
Less liquid base
Ice cubes

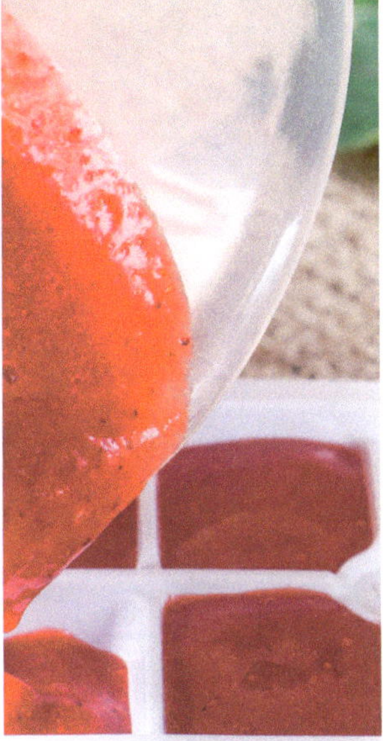

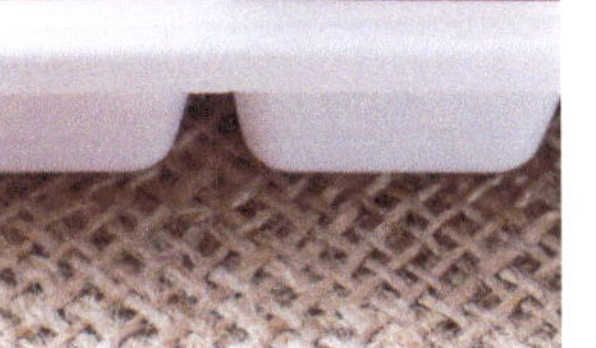

Consistency Adjustments:

For more liquid smoothies
Fresh fruit/vegetables, more liquid base

*Ice cubes made of frozen juice, plant based milk preferred over water

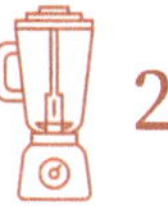

Strawberry Banana Cinnamon

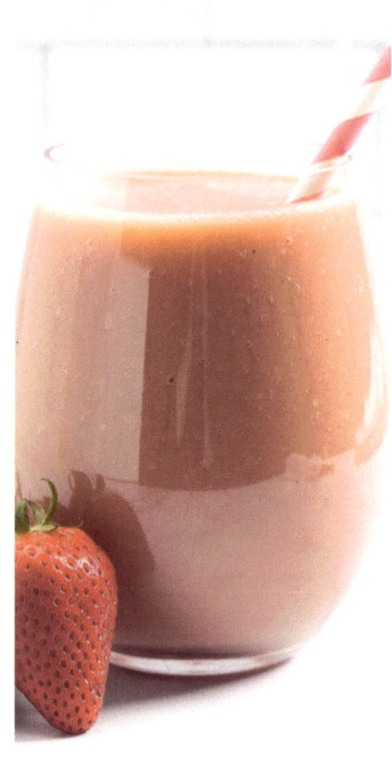

INGREDIENTS

1 C vanilla almond milk

1 C frozen strawberries (sliced)

1 frozen banana

medium ground cinnamon*

1 tablespoon of honey

INSTRUCTIONS

1. Add almond milk, frozen banana, and honey to blender.

Wait! Check your spice cap

2. Be sure you're on the sprinkle side. Now, lightly sprinkle a layer of cinnamon on top. Blend until smooth.

2. Add frozen strawberries. Blend until smooth.

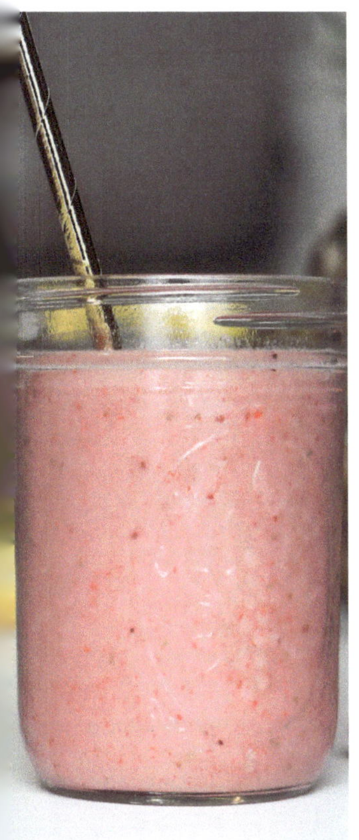

Zesty Strawberry

1. Add apple juice, lemon wedge, lime slices, & grapes to blender. Blend until smooth.

2. Add ⅔ cup of frozen strawberry slices. Blend until smooth.

3. Add the remaining ⅔ cup of frozen strawberry slices. Blend until smooth.

1C apple juice
⅔ frozen grapes

1 & ⅓ C strawberry slices frozen

1 lemon wedge (peeled)

2 slices of lime (peeled)

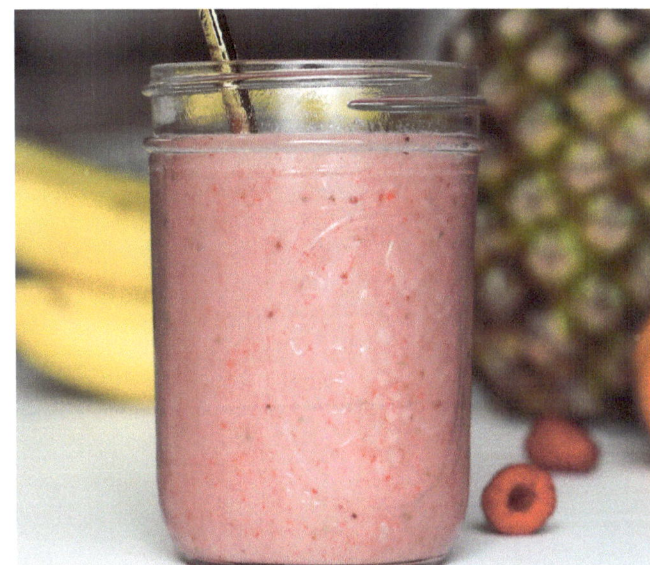

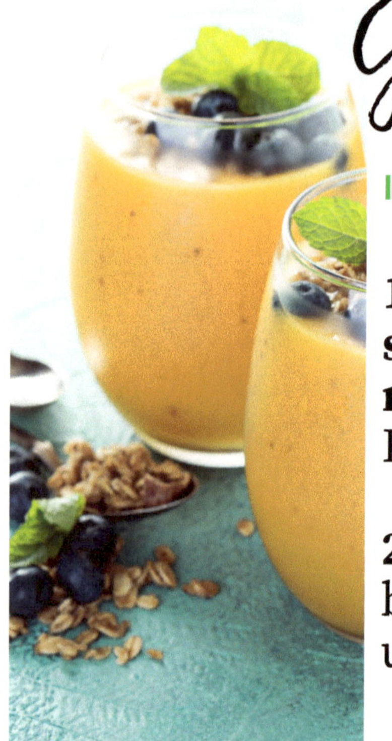

Greek Mango

1. Add apple juice, strawberry slice, and diced mango to blender.
Blend until smooth.

2. Add greek yogurt,
blending until color is uniformed.

INGREDIENTS

1C apple juice

1 C strawberry slices

 frozen

1 C vanilla, Greek

yogurt

1 ¼ C mango (diced)

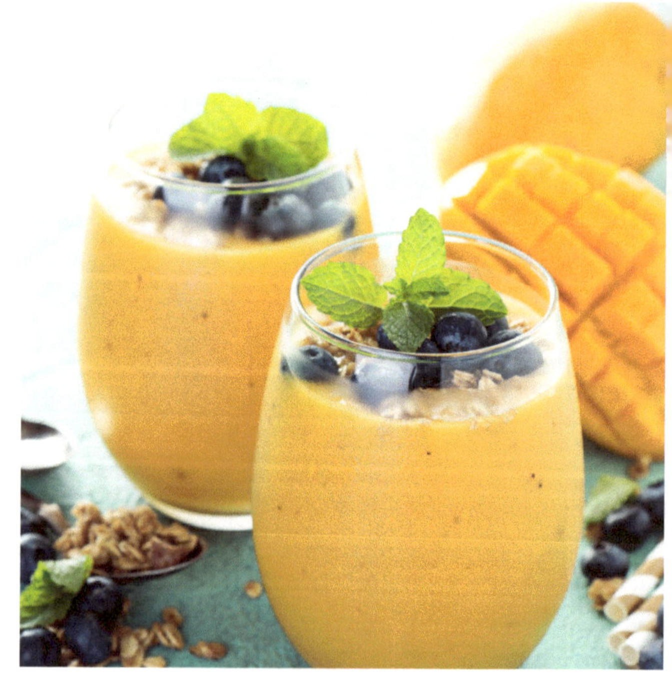

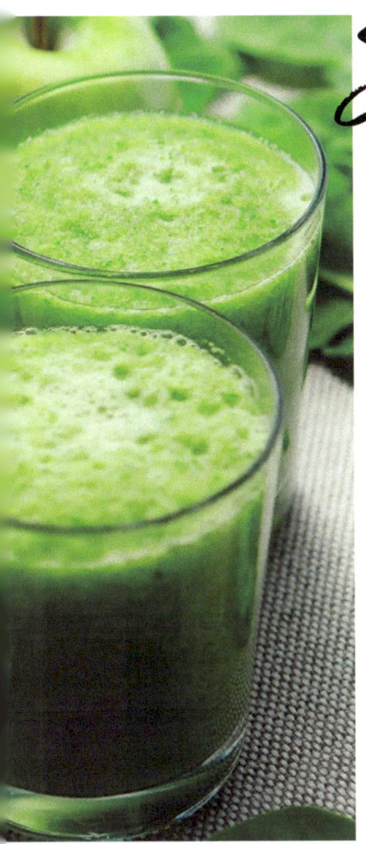

Sweet Greens

1. Pour grape juice & spinach into blender. Blend well.

2. Next, add apples only, blending until smooth.

3. Add frozen grapes and lemon. Blend until smooth.

4. Finally, add Greek yogurt & blend for about 2 seconds to maintain consistency.

INGREDIENTS

1 C spinach

½ C frozen, green grapes (seedless)

½ Granny Smith apple, large (sliced)

1 lemon slice, peeled

1 C white grape juice

1 C honey vanilla Greek yogurt

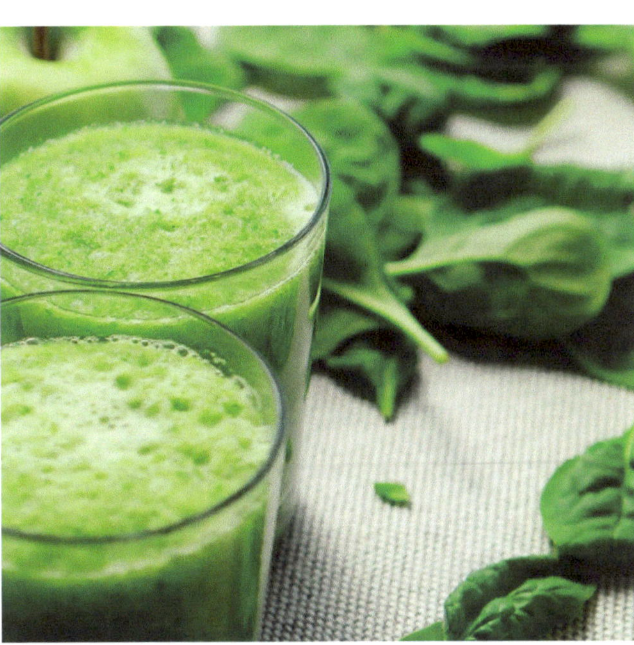

Mango Breeze

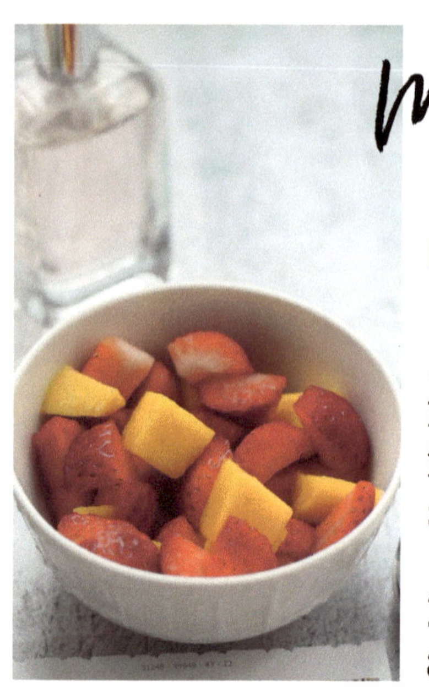

INGREDIENTS

1C apple juice

1 C of frozen

strawberries (sliced)

1, kiwi, frozen (sliced)

1 C diced mango

INSTRUCTIONS

1. Pour apple juice and frozen strawberries into blender. Blend until smooth.

2.Add frozen kiwi slices and diced mango. Blend until smooth.

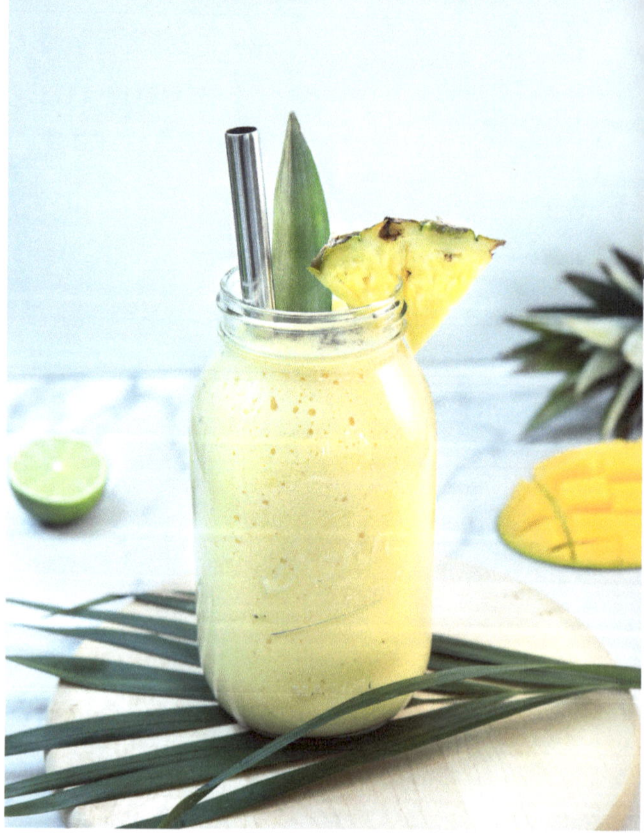

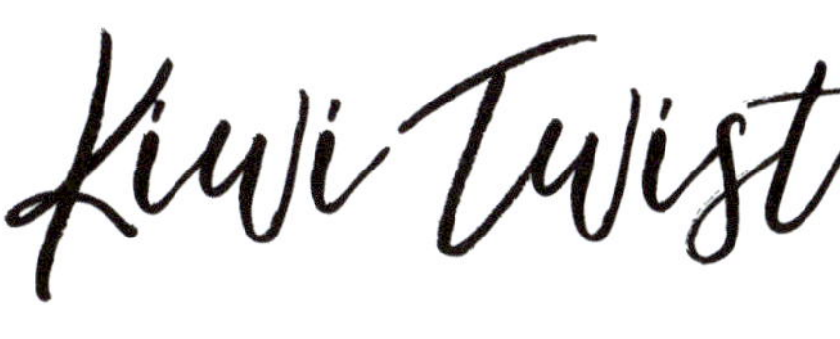
Kiwi Twist

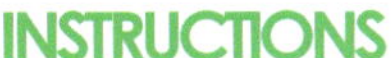

1. Pour apple juice and frozen grapes into blender. Blend until smooth.
2. Add frozen kiwi slices, blending until smooth.
3. Finally, add frozen strawberries. Blend until smooth.

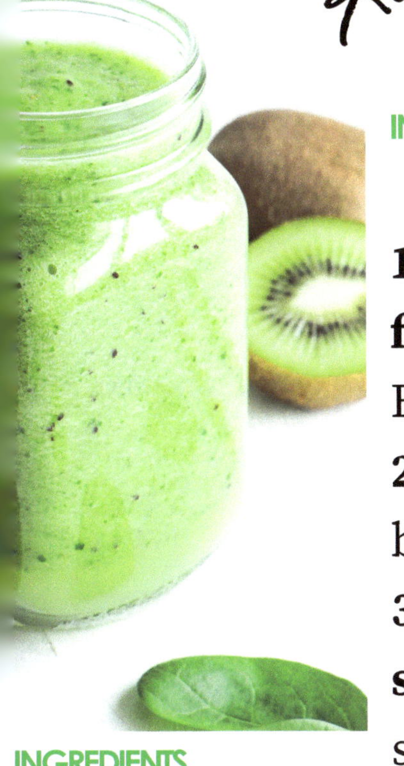

INGREDIENTS

1C apple juice
2 kiwis (peeled)
1/2 C frozen grapes (green)
1C frozen strawberries (sliced)

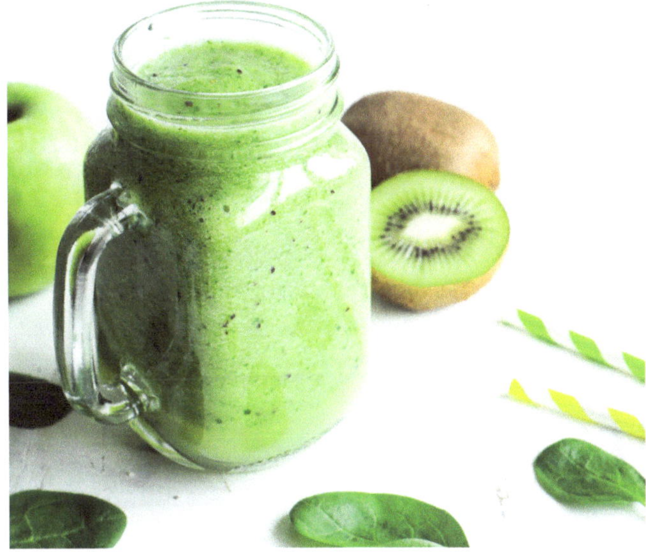

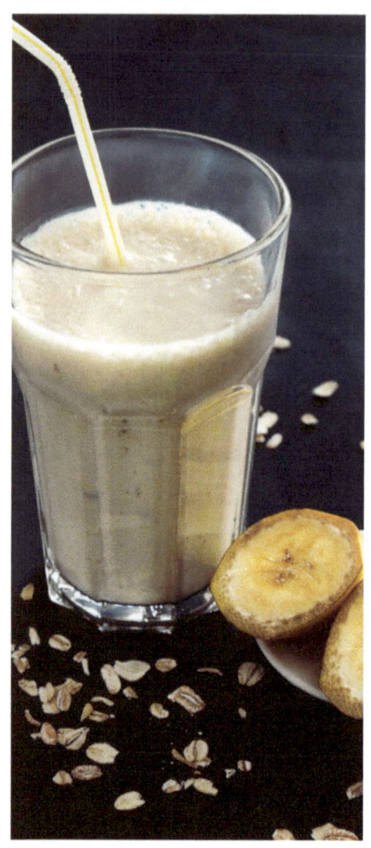

Peanut Butter Banana

1. Pour almond milk into blender

2. Add frozen banana

3. Add tablespoon of peanut butter

4. Blend until smooth

INGREDIENTS

1 peeled, frozen

banana (medium)

1 tablespoon of

peanut Butter

1 C almond milk

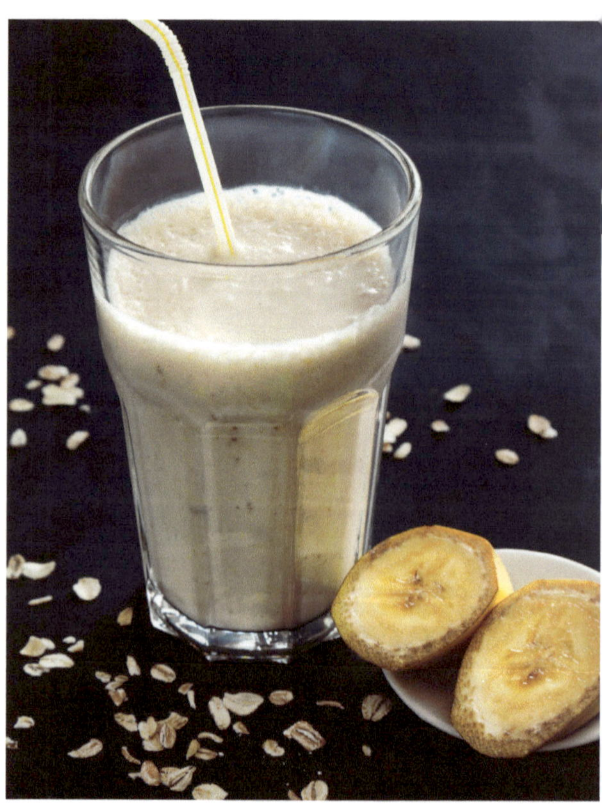

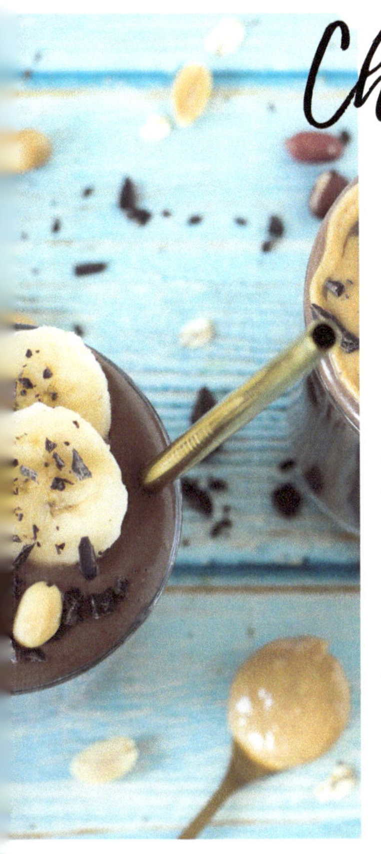

Chocolate Dipped Banana

1. **Pour almond milk into blender.**
2. **Add frozen banana.**
3. **Add cocoa powder.**
4. **Blend until smooth.**
5. **After smooth, sprinkle a light layer of ground cinnamon & pulse** blend for 3 seconds.

INGREDIENTS

1 1/2 medium, frozen bananas (peeled)

1/8 teaspoon of cocoa powder

ground cinnamon

1 C almond milk

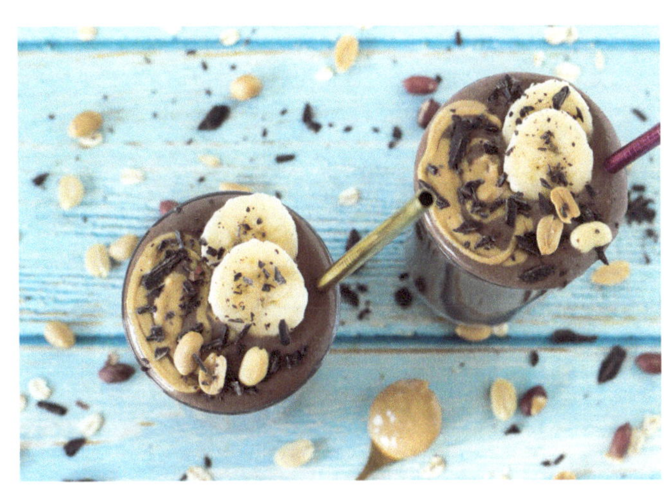

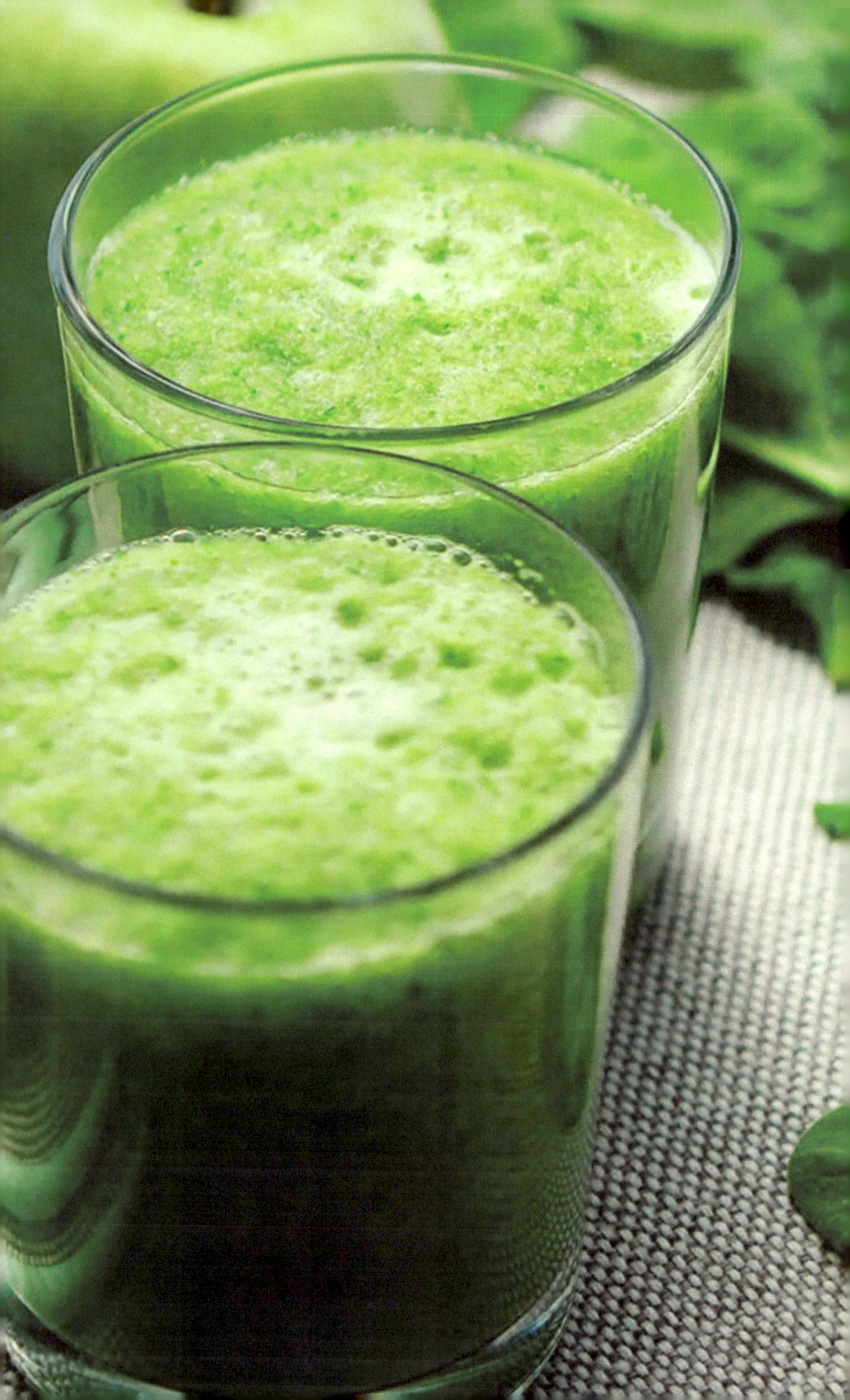

References

Centers for Disease Control and Prevention, U.S. Department of Health and Human Services. "The Problem 1/2 1 in 6 - Centers for Disease Control and Prevention." VITAMIN & MINERAL NUTRITION FOR HEALTHY GROWTH AND DEVELOPMENT, Apr. 2020, www.cdc.gov/nutrition/micronutrient-malnutrition/about-micronutrients/pdfs/MicronutrientFactsheet-April2020-508.pdf.

U.S. Food and Drug Administration. "Https://Www.Natrol-Llc.Com/FDA-Vitamin-Mineral-Chart.Pdf." Interactive Nutrition Facts Label, Oct. 2021, www.accessdata.fda.gov/scripts/interactivenutritionfactslabel/assets/InteractiveNFL_Vitamins&MineralsChart_October2021.pdf.

National Mango Board. "Mango Nutrition Facts Label." Mango.Org, 1 Aug. 2022, www.mango.org/mango-nutrition-facts-label/.

U.S. Department of Agriculture. "Fooddata Central Search Results." FoodData Central, fdc.nal.usda.gov/fdc-app.html#/. Accessed 22 May 2023.

U.S. Department of Health & Human Services. "Office of Dietary Supplements (ODS)." NIH Office of Dietary Supplements, ods.od.nih.gov/. Accessed 22 May 2023.

Mindell, Earl. The Vitamins & Minerals Bible: Miracle Foods to Boost Your Health. Hamlyn, 2017.

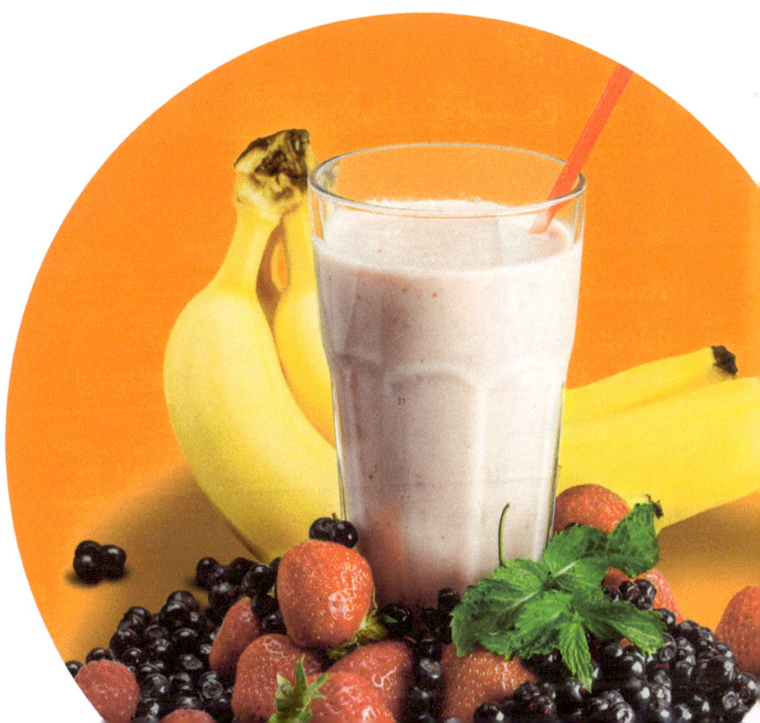

Photograhy

Shutter Stock

1668309727-huge
shutterstock_173275574
shutterstock_283259678
shutterstock_283340090
shutterstock_396837793
shutterstock_406827097
shutterstock_444839779
shutterstock_477268198
shutterstock_664613644
shutterstock_667611496
shutterstock_1253619040
shutterstock_1915529911
shutterstock_1927073573
shutterstock_1934663255
shutterstock_2123401991
shutterstock_2196946997
shutterstock_2221039761

Adobe Stock

AdobeStock_271682776
frustratedwoman
AdobeStock_344731861

Unsplash

andrijana-bozic-Oxh-t-EhNC4-unsplash
element5-digital-kxW731QLajM-unsplash
jugoslocos-GHsf8ny3LF0-unsplash
keesha-s-kitchen-UyAns1_w6YU-unsplash
elena-leya-JfWhrxbmF-U-unsplash

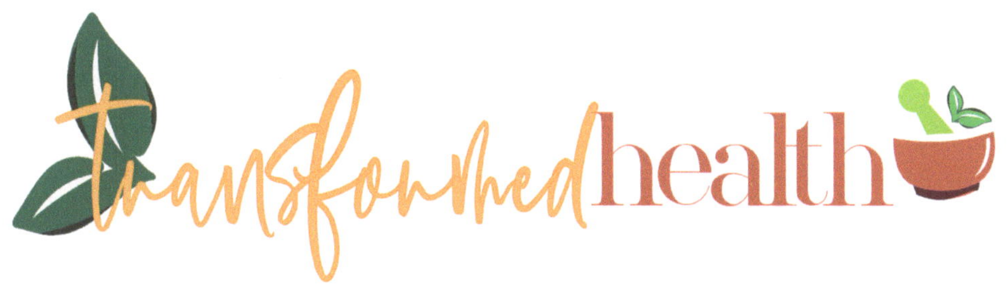

Don't forget to book your complimentary consult 'Tea with Dr. Bri' for an introductory health chat. Visit **transformedhealth.org** to book.

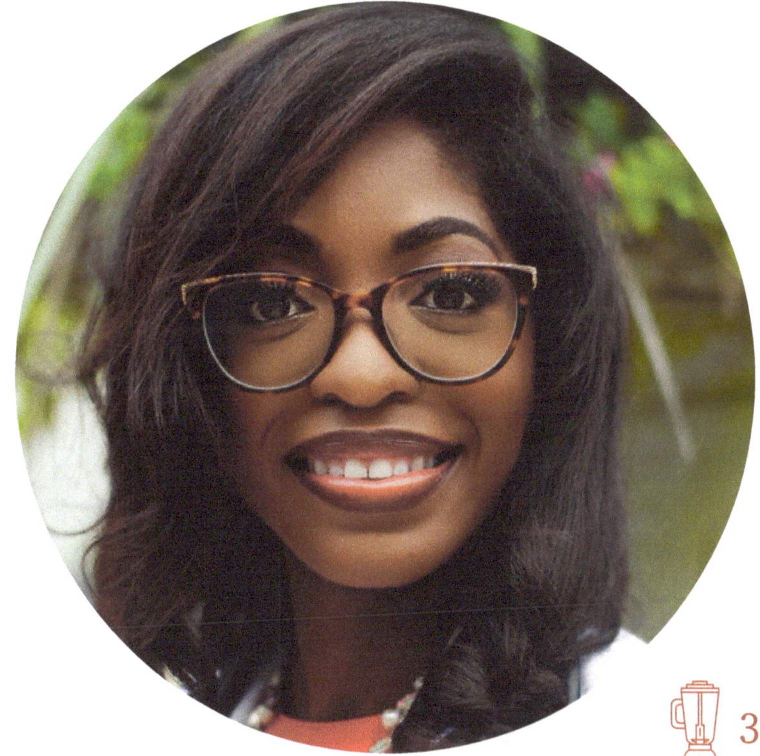